Mediterranean Diet Crash-Course

*An Effective Guide Step-By-Step Guide For Beginners
To Eat Well And Stay Healthy With These
Mediterranean Recipes*

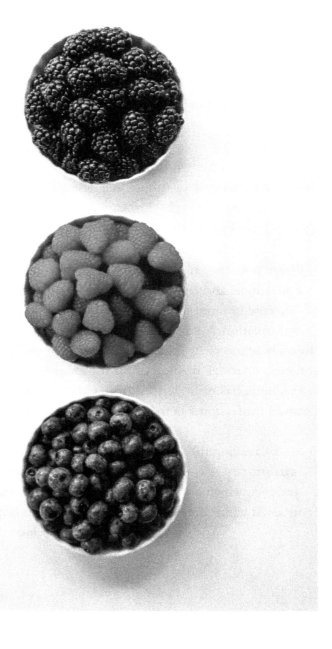

Table of Contents

CHAPTER 5: TASTY FIRST COURSES TO BRING TO YOUR TABLE .. 44

CHAPTER 6: HERE ARE THE MAIN COURSES OF MEAT THAT WILL MAKE YOU THE MASTER CHEF OF YOUR CIRCLE OF FRIENDS 60

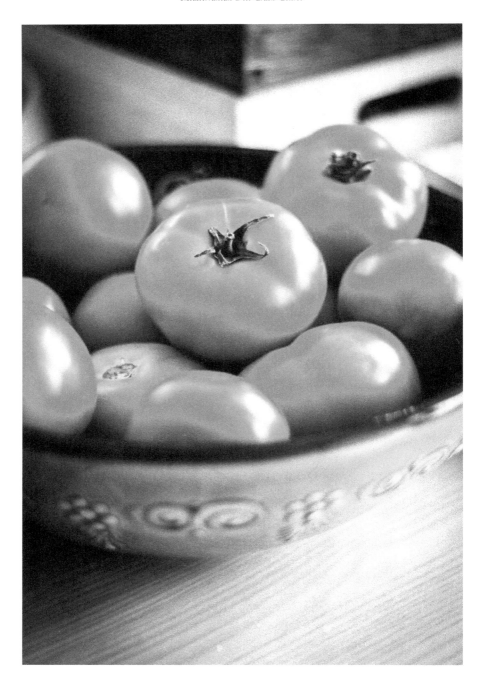

Introduction

The Mediterranean diet is a diet that has been proven to help prevent several types of cancer and prevent cardiovascular and heart problems. This diet has been adopted all over Italy, Greece, France, and Spain. The Mediterranean diet is healthier than the American diet as it is provided by the government because it lacks animal fat, cholesterol, and high glycemic foods. The diet focuses more on fresh fruits and vegetables, not junk food and processed food. The Mediterranean diet has the right number of calories, providing people with plenty of energy. In addition to daily physical activities, the diet will improve your overall health and lower the risk of living the American lifestyle.

Once the diet has been adopted into one's life on a permanent basis, they are still left with the permanent problem of obesity and poor health. This is because people do not follow the diet; they just use it as a temporary change after neck surgery, heart attack, or to lose weight. The only way one can successfully adopt the Mediterranean diet and lifestyle is to live for a longer period of time by making the diet and lifestyle permanent.

In terms of overcoming the obstacles that face those who choose to follow the Mediterranean diet, one must sacrifice many foods that taste sweet and common throughout the United States. In order to overcome these food habits, one must substitute common sweet foods with healthier options such as nuts or dried fruits. Furthermore, to overcome the fact that the Mediterranean diet lacks seasonal fresh fruits and vegetables, one must substitute them with unhealthy items such as processed foods.

The second problem of obesity and poor health is the exercises that one must engage in daily in order to lose weight successfully. Once again, it is hard for someone to stay motivated to stay active when it is not enjoyable. For example, running is boring; it is just not fun for children or adults. However, there are many enjoyable physical activities to keep the body fit and healthy.

My favorite physical activity to stay in shape is a hiking and rock climbing. The adrenaline rush is awesome, but even if one does not enjoy outdoor activities, there are other ways to stay fit.

The Mediterranean diet is full of never-ending varieties of healthy, fresh, and delicious foods. However, there is more of an emphasis on certain types of foods; nothing is excluded. People who try a Mediterranean diet can enjoy the dishes they love while also learning to appreciate how good the freshest, healthiest foods can be.

Transitioning into the Mediterranean diet is mainly about bracing yourself for a new way of eating, adapting your attitude toward food into one of joyful expectation and appreciation of good meals and good company. It's like a mindset as anything else, so you'll want to make your environment unite so you can quickly adapt to the lifestyle in the Mediterranean way.

In conclusion, obesity and poor health are two problems that have plagued the world for a long time now. Obesity is characterized by an excessive accumulation of body fat. This excessive accumulation of fat may cause heart disease, diabetes, and even cancer. The Mediterranean diet and lifestyle, coupled with physical activities, are required to overcome obesity and poor health.

CHAPTER 1:

Particular Aspects of the Mediterranean Diet Compared to Other Types of Diets

Benefits of the Mediterranean Diet

1. **Boosts Your Brain Health.** Preserve memory and prevent cognitive decline by following a Mediterranean diet that will limit processed foods, refined bread, and red meats. Have a glass of wine versus hard liquor.

2. **Improves Poor Eyesight.** Older individuals suffer from poor eyesight, but in many cases, the Mediterranean diet has provided notable improvement. An Australian Center for Eye Research discovered that the individuals who consumed a minimum of 100 ml (0.42 cup) of olive oil weekly were almost 50% less likely to develop macular degeneration versus those who ate less than one ml each week.

3. **Helps to Reduce the Risk of Heart Disease.** The New England Journal of Medicine provided evidence in 2013 from a randomized clinical trial. The trial was implemented in Spain, whereas individuals did not have cardiovascular disease at enrollment but were in the 'high risk' category. The incidence of major cardiovascular events was reduced by the Mediterranean diet that was supplemented with extra-virgin olive oil or nuts. In one study, men who consumed fish in this manner reduced the risk by 23% of death from heart disease.

4. **The Risk of Alzheimer's Disease Is Reduced.** In 2018, the journal Neurology studied 70 brain scans of individuals who had no signs of dementia at the onset. They followed the eating patterns in a two-year study resulting in individuals who were on the Med diet had a lesser increase of the depots and reduced energy use — potentially signaling risk for Alzheimer's.

5. **Helps Lessen the Risk of Some Types of Cancer.** According to the results of a group study, the diet is associated with a lessened risk of stomach cancer (gastric adenocarcinoma).

6. **Decreases Risks for Type 2 Diabetes.** It can help stabilize blood sugar while protecting against type 2 diabetes with its low-carb elements. The Med diet maintains a richness in fiber, which will digest slowly while preventing variances in your blood sugar. It also can help you maintain a healthier weight, which is another trigger for diabetes.

7. **Suggests Improvement for Those with Parkinson's Disease.** By consuming foods on the Mediterranean diet, you add high levels of antioxidants that can prevent your body from undergoing oxidative stress, which is a damaging process that will attack your cells. The menu plan can reduce your risk factors in half.

Mediterranean Diet Pyramid

The Mediterranean Diet Pyramid is a nutritional guide developed by the World Health Organization, Harvard School of Public Health, and Old ways Preservation Trust in 1993. It is a visual tool that summarizes the Mediterranean diet, suggested eating patterns, and guides how frequently specific mechanisms should be eaten. It allows you to break healthy eating habits and not overfill yourself with too many calories.

- **Olive Oil, Fruits, Vegetables, Whole Grains, Legumes, Beans, Nuts & Seeds, Spices & Herbs**. These foods form the Mediterranean pyramid base. If you did observe, you would notice that these are mostly from plant sources. You should try and include a few variations of these items into each meal you eat. Olive oil should be the primary fat in cooking your dishes and endeavor to replace any other butter or cooking oil you may have been using to cook.

- **Fish & Seafood**. These are essential staples of the Mediterranean diet that should be consumed often as a protein source. You would want to include these in your diet at least two times a week. Try new varieties of fish, either frozen or fresh. Also, incorporate seafood like mussels, crab, and shrimp into your diet. Canned tuna is also great to include on sandwiches or toss in a salad with fresh vegetables.

- **Cheese, Yogurt, Eggs & Poultry**. These ingredients should be consumed in more moderate amounts. Depending on the food, they should be used sparingly throughout the week. Keep in

11

mind that if you are using eggs in baking or cooking, they will also be counted in your weekly limit. You would want to stick to more healthy cheese like Parmesan, ricotta, or feta that you can add a topping or garnish on your dishes.

- **Red Meat & Sweets**. These items are going to be consumed less frequently. If you are going to eat them, you need to consume only small quantities, most preferably lean meat versions with less fat when possible. Most studies recommend a maximum of 12 to 16 ounces per month. To add more variety to your diet, you can still have red meat occasionally, but you would want to reduce how often you have it. It is essential to limit its intake because of all the health concerns of sugar and red meat. The Mediterranean diet improves cardiovascular health and reduces blood pressure, while red meat tends to be dangerous to your cardiovascular system. The Greece population ate very little red meat and instead had fish or seafood as their main protein source.

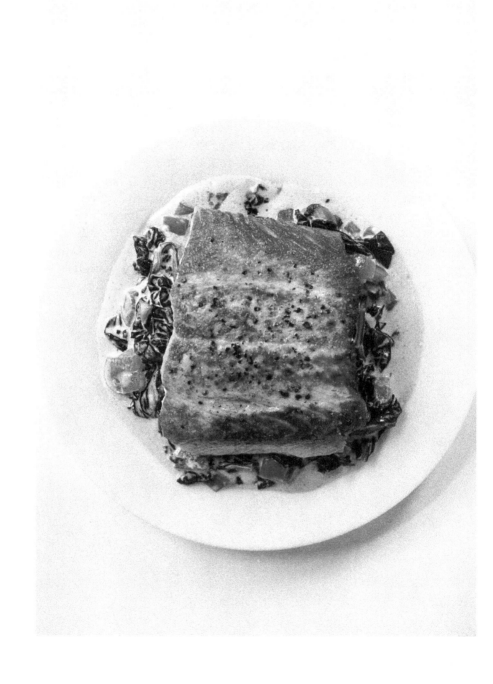

CHAPTER 2:

Diet Associated with Healthy Exercise and Healthy Habits

The Mediterranean diet is a lifestyle more than a mere diet. It's safe to say the Mediterranean diet is both a brain-friendly and a body-friendly diet because it preserves and keeps them balanced in their respective ways. Therefore, as long as you follow this Mediterranean diet and continue to enrich your lifestyle with the balanced meal options it provides, you are assured of leading a safe and wonderful life without diseases hiding nearby.

In fact, the Italian Mediterranean diet is one of the very first and most popular diets in the world today, as it has been proven to be a great, healthy diet. Indeed, the Italian Mediterranean diet changes the way people view dieting and adhering to a strict diet plan. Be as it may, there is a lot more to the diet plan than merely following a strict diet plan, and sticking to it will undoubtedly be enough to keep one fit and healthy.

The dietary pattern is connected through reductions of all-cause mortality in observational studies. There is also some indication that the Mediterranean diet decreases the risk of heart failure and early death; that is why the American Medical Association and the (AHA) American Heart Association suggest this diet.

Though there are many opposing views on the Mediterranean diet, some controversy over some sources says that the Italian Mediterranean diet is actually not that great because there are numerous other diets similar in style to that.

It has been proven to be an excellent way of maintaining health and living a long, healthy life. Still, the Italian Mediterranean diet is an excellent way of living and has been proven to produce great results. It is undoubtedly a great diet plan to follow. The Italian Mediterranean diet can also create long-term effects in keeping one's heart-healthy and body functioning at optimum levels.

Tips to Start off

The Mediterranean diet is a straightforward, easy to follow, and delicious diet, but you need a bit of preparation. Preparing for the Mediterranean diet is largely about preparing yourself for a new way of eating and adjusting your attitude toward food into one of joyful expectation and appreciation of good meals and good company. There are a few things to make your transition to the diet easier and effortless.

Ease Your Way Into More Healthful Eating

Before starting the diet, it can be helpful to spend a week or two cutting back on the least healthful foods that you are currently eating. You might start with fast food or eliminate cream-based sauces and soups. You can begin by cutting back on processed foods like frozen meals, boxed dinners, and chips. Some other things to start trimming might be sodas, coffee with a lot of sugar, and milk. You should lower butter and cut out red meats such as lamb, beef, and pork.

Start Thinking About What You'll Be Eating

Just like planning for a vacation, you need to plan your diet. Go through the list of foods you need to eat on the Mediterranean diet and get recipes and meal ideas.

Gather What You'll Need

Everything in the Mediterranean diet is easily found at farmers' markets, grocery stores, and seafood shops. Find out where your local farmers' markets are, and spend a leisurely morning checking out what is available. Talk to the farmers about what they harvest and when. Building relationships with those vendors can lead to getting special deals and the best selection.

You can join the CSA (Community Supported Agriculture) farm nearby. CSA farms are small farms that sell subscription packages of whatever they're growing that season.

For a moderate seasonal or weekly fee, the farm will supply you with enough of that week's harvest to feed your whole family. Freshness is important when following the Mediterranean diet. Joining a CSA is a great way to enjoy the freshness and peak flavor that is so important to the Mediterranean diet. The same is true for your local seafood market and butcher shop.

Find out who's selling the freshest, most healthful meats and seafood and buy from them. When you're ready to start, create a shopping list and get as many of your ingredients from your new sources as you can.

Plan Your Week

Planning ahead is essential to success. The diet is heavily plant-based, and you need to load up on fresh fruits, vegetables, and herbs each week. By keeping your pantry stocked with whole grains like whole-wheat pasta, polenta, dried or canned beans and legumes, olive oil, and even some canned vegetables and fish, you can be sure that you'll always have the ingredients for a healthy meal.

Adjust Your Portions

The idea behind the Mediterranean diet is to make up the bulk of your diet with plant-based foods like fruits, vegetables, whole grains, beans, and nuts. Foods like cheese, meat, and sweets are allowed, but they are consumed only occasionally and in small portions.

One way to ensure that you're eating enough plant-based foods while following the Mediterranean diet is to fill half your plate with vegetables and fruit, then fill one-quarter with whole grains, and the last quarter your plate with protein such as beans, fish, shellfish, or poultry.

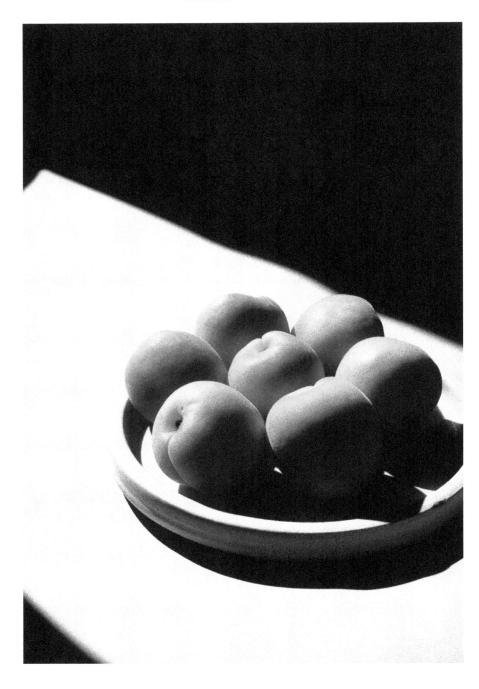

CHAPTER 3:

Recipes for an Energetic and Tasty Breakfast

1. Avocado Egg Scramble

Preparation Time: 8 minutes

Cooking Time: 15 minutes

Servings: 4

Ingredients:

- Four eggs, beaten
- One white onion, diced
- One tablespoon avocado oil
- One avocado, finely chopped

- ½ teaspoon chili flakes

- 1 oz Cheddar cheese, shredded

- ½ teaspoon salt

- One tablespoon fresh parsley

Directions:

1. Pour avocado oil into the skillet and bring it to a boil.

2. Then add diced onion and roast it until it is light brown.

3. Meanwhile, mix up together chili flakes, beaten eggs, and salt.

4. Pour the egg mixture over the cooked onion and cook the mixture for 1 minute over medium heat.

5. After this, scramble the eggs well with the help of the fork or spatula. Cook the eggs until they are solid but soft.

6. After this, add chopped avocado and shredded cheese.

7. Stir the scrambled well and transfer in the serving plates.

8. Sprinkle the meal with fresh parsley.

Nutrition:

- Calories: 236

- Fat: 20.1 g

- Fiber: 4 g

- Carbs: 7.4 g

- Protein: 8.6 g

2.   Breakfast Tostadas

Preparation Time: 15 minutes

Cooking Time: 6 minutes

Servings: 6

Ingredients:

- ½ white onion, diced

- One tomato, chopped

- One cucumber, chopped

- One tablespoon fresh cilantro, chopped

- ½ jalapeno pepper, chopped

- One tablespoon lime juice

- Six corn tortillas

- One tablespoon canola oil

- 2 oz Cheddar cheese, shredded

- ½ cup white beans, canned, drained

- Six eggs

- ½ teaspoon butter

- ½ teaspoon Sea salt

Directions:

1. Make Pico de Gallo: In the salad bowl, combine diced white onion, tomato, cucumber, fresh cilantro, and jalapeno pepper.

2. Then add lime juice and a ½ tablespoon of canola oil. Mix up the mixture well. Pico de Gallo is cooked.

3. After this, preheat the oven to 390F.

4. Line the tray with baking paper.

5. Arrange the corn tortillas on the baking paper and brush with the remaining canola oil from both sides.

6. Bake the tortillas for 10 minutes or wait until they start to be crunchy.

7. Chill the cooked crunchy tortillas well.

8. Meanwhile, toss the butter in the skillet.

9. Crack the eggs in the melted butter and sprinkle them with sea salt.

10. Fry the eggs until the egg whites become white (cooked). Approximately 3-5 minutes over medium heat.

11. After this, mash the beans until you get a puree texture.

12. Spread the bean puree on the corn tortillas.

13. Add fried eggs.

14. Then top the eggs with Pico de Gallo and shredded Cheddar cheese.

Nutrition:

- Calories: 246

- Fat: 11.1 g

- Fiber: 4.7 g

- Carbs: 24.5 g

- Protein: 13.7 g

3. Parmesan Omelet

Preparation Time: 5 minutes

Cooking Time: 10 minutes

Servings: 2

Ingredients:

- One tablespoon cream cheese

- Two eggs, beaten

- ¼ teaspoon paprika

- ½ teaspoon dried oregano

- ¼ teaspoon dried dill

- 1 oz Parmesan, grated

- One teaspoon coconut oil

Directions:

1. Mix up together cream cheese with eggs, dried oregano, and dill.

2. Put coconut oil in the frypan and heat it until it coats all the skillet.

3. Then pour the egg mixture into the skillet and flatten it.

4. Add grated Parmesan and close the lid.

5. Cook the omelet for 10 minutes over low heat.

6. Then transfer the cooked omelet to the serving plate and sprinkle with paprika.

Nutrition:

- Calories: 148

- Fat: 11.5 g

- Fiber: 0.3 g

- Carbs: 1.4 g

- Protein: 10.6 g

4.   Menemen

Preparation Time: 6 minutes

Cooking Time: 15 minutes

Servings: 4

Ingredients:

- Two tomatoes, chopped

- Two eggs, beaten

- One bell pepper, chopped

- One teaspoon tomato paste

- ¼ cup of water

- One teaspoon butter

- ½ white onion, diced

- ½ teaspoon chili flakes

- 1/3 teaspoon sea salt

Directions:

1. Put butter in the pan and thaw it.

2. Add bell pepper and cook it for 3 minutes over medium heat. Stir it from time to time.

3. After this, add diced onion and cook it for 2 minutes more.

4. Stir the vegetables and add tomatoes.

5. Cook them for 5 minutes with medium-low heat.

6. Then add water and tomato paste. Stir well.

7. Add beaten eggs, chili flakes, and sea salt.

8. Stir well and cook the menemen for 4 minutes over medium-low heat.

9. The cooked meal should be half runny.

Nutrition:

- Calories: 67 Fat: 3.4 g

- Fiber: 1.5 g

- Carbs: 6.4 g

- Protein: 3.8 g

5.   Morning Pizza with Sprouts

Preparation Time: 15 minutes **Cooking Time:** 20 minutes

Servings: 6

Ingredients:

- ½ cup wheat flour, whole grain

- Two tablespoons butter, softened

- ¼ teaspoon baking powder

- ¾ teaspoon salt

- 5 oz chicken fillet, boiled

- 2 oz Cheddar cheese, shredded

- One teaspoon tomato sauce

- 1 oz bean sprouts

Directions:

1. Make the pizza crust: Mix up together wheat flour, butter, baking powder, and salt. Knead the soft and non-sticky dough. Add more wheat flour if needed.

2. Leave the dough for 10 minutes to chill.

3. Then place the dough on the baking paper. Cover it with the second baking paper sheet.

4. Roll up the dough with the help of the rolling pin to get the round pizza crust.

5. After this, remove the upper baking paper sheet.

6. Transfer the pizza crust to the tray.

7. Spread the crust with tomato sauce.

8. Then shred the chicken fillet and arrange it over the pizza crust. Add shredded Cheddar cheese.

9. Bake the pizza for 20 minutes at 355F.

10. Then top the cooked pizza with bean sprouts and slice it into servings.

Nutrition:

- Calories: 157 Fat: 8.8 g Fiber: 0.3 g

- Carbs: 8.4 g Protein: 10.5 g

6. Banana Quinoa

Preparation Time: 10 minutes

Cooking Time: 12 minutes

Servings: 4

Ingredients:

- 1 cup quinoa

- 2 cup milk

- One teaspoon vanilla extract

- One teaspoon honey

- Two bananas, sliced

- ¼ teaspoon ground cinnamon

Directions:

1. Pour milk into the saucepan and add quinoa.

2. Close the lid and cook it over medium heat for 12 minutes or until quinoa will absorb all liquid.

3. Then chill the quinoa for 10-15 minutes and place in the serving mason jars.

4. Add honey, vanilla extract, and ground cinnamon.

5. Stir well.

6. Top quinoa with banana and stir it before serving.

Nutrition:

- Calories: 279

- Fat: 5.3 g

- Fiber: 4.6 g

- Carbs: 48.4 g

- Protein: 10.7 g

CHAPTER 4:

Snack Recipes That Drive Young and Old Alike Crazy

7.   Figs with Mascarpone and Honey

Preparation Time: 5 minutes

Cooking Time: 5 minutes

Servings: 4

Ingredients:

- 1/3 cup walnuts, chopped

- Eight fresh figs halved

- ¼ cup mascarpone cheese

- One tablespoon honey

- ¼ teaspoon flaked sea salt

Directions:

1. In a frypan with medium heat, toast the walnuts, often stirring, for 3 to 5 minutes.

2. Arrange the figs cut-side up on a plate or platter. Using your finger, create a small depression in each fig's cut side and fill with mascarpone cheese. Sprinkle with a bit of the walnut, drizzle with the honey, and add a tiny pinch of sea salt.

Nutrition:

- Calories: 200

- Total Fat: 13g

- Cholesterol: 18mg

- Total Carbohydrates: 24g

- Protein: 3g

8.   Pistachio-Stuffed Dates

Preparation Time: 10 minutes **Cooking Time:** 0 minutes

Servings: 4

Ingredients:

- ½ cup unsalted pistachios shelled

- ¼ teaspoon kosher salt

- 8 Medjool dates, pitted

Directions:

1. In a food processor, add the salt and pistachios. Process until combined to chunky nut butter, 3 to 5 minutes.

2. Split open the dates and spoon the pistachio nut butter into each half.

Nutrition:

- Calories: 220 Total Fat: 7g Cholesterol: 0mg

- Total Carbohydrates: 41g Protein: 4g

9.   Portable Packed Picnic Pieces

Preparation Time: 10 minutes

Cooking Time: 0 minutes

Servings: 1

Ingredients:

- 1-slice of whole-wheat bread, cut into bite-size pieces

- 10-pcs cherry tomatoes

- ¼-oz. aged cheese, sliced

- 6-pcs oil-cured olives

Directions:

1. Pack each of the ingredients in a portable container to serve you while snacking on the go.

Nutrition:

- Calories: 197 Total Fats: 9g

- Fiber: 4g Carbohydrates: 22g

- Protein: 7g

10. Naturally Nutty & Buttery Banana Bowl

Preparation Time: 5 minutes

Cooking Time: 0 minutes

Servings: 4

Ingredients:

- 4-cups vanilla Greek yogurt

- 2-pcs medium-sized bananas, sliced

- ¼-cup creamy and natural peanut butter

- 1-tsp ground nutmeg

- ¼-cup flaxseed meal

Directions:

1. Divide the yogurt equally between four serving bowls.
   Top each yogurt bowl with the banana slices.

2. Put the peanut butter inside a microwave-safe bowl.
   Melt the peanut butter in your microwave for 40

seconds. Drizzle one tablespoon of the melted peanut butter over the bananas for each bowl.

3. To serve, sprinkle over with the ground nutmeg and flax-seed meal.

Nutrition:

- Calories: 370

- Total Fats: 10.6g

- Fiber: 4.7g

- Carbohydrates: 47.7g

- Protein: 22.7g

11. Brussels Sprouts with Pistachios

Preparation Time: 15 minutes **Cooking Time:** 15 minutes

Servings: 4

Ingredients:

- 1-pound Brussels sprouts, tough bottoms trimmed, halved lengthwise

- Four shallots, peeled and quartered

- One tablespoon extra-virgin olive oil

- Sea salt

- Freshly ground black pepper

- ½ cup chopped roasted pistachios

- Zest of ½ lemon

- Juice of ½ lemon

Directions:

1. Preheat the oven to 400°F.

2. In a bowl, toss the Brussels sprouts and shallots with the olive oil until well coated.

3. Season with sea salt and pepper, and then spread the vegetables evenly on the sheet.

4. Bake for 15 minutes, or until tender and lightly caramelized.

5. Take away from the oven and transfer to a serving bowl.

6. Toss with the pistachios, lemon zest, and lemon juice. Serve warm.

Nutrition:

- Calories: 126

- Total Fat: 7g

- Saturated Fat: 1g

- Carbohydrates: 14g Fiber: 5g

- Protein: 6g

12.　Roasted Parmesan Broccoli

Preparation Time: 10 minutes

Cooking Time: 10 minutes

Servings: 4

Ingredients:

- Two heads broccoli, cut into small florets

- Two tablespoons extra-virgin olive oil

- Two teaspoons minced garlic

- Zest of 1 lemon

- Juice of 1 lemon

- Pinch sea salt

- ½ cup grated Parmesan cheese

Directions:

1. Preheat the oven to 400°F.

2. Lightly grease a baking sheet using olive oil and set it aside.

3. In a large bowl, toss the broccoli with two tablespoons of olive oil, garlic, lemon zest, lemon juice, and sea salt

4. Spread the combination on the baking sheet in a single layer and sprinkle with the Parmesan cheese.

5. Bake for about 10 minutes, or until tender. Transfer the broccoli to a serving dish and serve.

Nutrition:

- Calories: 154

- Total Fat: 11g

- Saturated Fat: 3g

- Carbohydrates: 10g

- Fiber: 4

- Protein: 9g

13. Cucumber Hummus Sandwiches

Preparation Time: 5 minutes

Cooking Time: 0 minutes

Servings: 1

Ingredients:

- 10 round slices of cucumber

- Five teaspoons hummus

Directions:

1. Add one teaspoon hummus to one slice of cucumber.

2. Top with another slice and serve.

Nutrition:

- Calories: 54

- Fat: 21g

- Total Carbs: 7g

- Protein: 2g

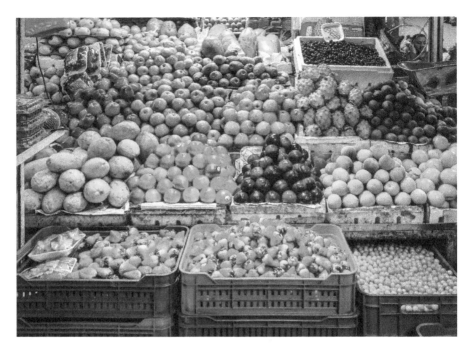

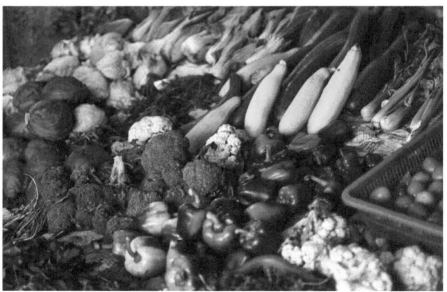

CHAPTER 5:

Tasty First Courses to Bring to Your Table

14. Italian Mac & Cheese

Preparation Time: 10 minutes

Cooking Time: 6 minutes

Servings: 4

Ingredients:

- 1 lb. whole grain pasta

- 2 tsp Italian seasoning

- 1 ½ tsp garlic powder

- 1 ½ tsp onion powder

- 1 cup sour cream

- 4 cups of water

- 4 oz parmesan cheese, shredded

- 12 oz ricotta cheese

- Pepper

- Salt

Directions:

1. Add all the ingredients except ricotta cheese into the inner pot of the instant pot and stir well.

2. Cook on high for 6 minutes. Add ricotta cheese and stir well and serve.

Nutrition:

- Calories: 388 Fat: 25.8 g

- Carbohydrates: 18.1 g

- Sugar: 4 g

- Protein: 22.8 g

- Cholesterol: 74 mg

15. Italian Chicken Pasta

Preparation Time: 10 minutes

Cooking Time: 9 minutes

Servings: 8

Ingredients:

- 1 lb. chicken breast, skinless, boneless, and cut into chunks

- ½ cup cream cheese

- 1 cup mozzarella cheese, shredded

- 1 ½ tsp Italian seasoning

- 1 tsp garlic, minced

- 1 cup mushrooms, diced

- ½ onion, diced

- 2 tomatoes, diced

- 2 cups of water

- 16 oz whole wheat penne pasta

- Pepper

- Salt

Directions:

1. Add all the ingredients except cheeses into the inner pot of the instant pot and stir well.

2. Cook on high for 9 minutes. Add cheeses and stir well and serve.

Nutrition:

- Calories: 328

- Fat: 8.5 g

- Carbohydrates: 42.7 g

- Sugar: 1.4 g

- Protein: 23.7 g

- Cholesterol: 55 mg

16.   Spinach Pesto Pasta

Preparation Time: 10 minutes

Cooking Time: 10 minutes

Servings: 4

Ingredients:

- 8 oz whole-grain pasta

- 1/3 cup mozzarella cheese, grated

- ½ cup pesto

- 5 oz fresh spinach

- 1 3/4 cup water

- 8 oz mushrooms, chopped

- 1 tbsp olive oil Pepper Salt

Directions:

1. Warm oil into the pot and sauté mushrooms for 5 minutes.

2. Add water and pasta and stir well. Set on high and cook for 5 minutes. Stir in the remaining ingredients and serve.

Nutrition:

- Calories: 213

- Fat: 17.3 g

- Carbohydrates: 9.5 g

- Sugar: 4.5 g

- Protein: 7.4 g

- Cholesterol: 9 mg

17. Fiber Packed Chicken Rice

Preparation Time: 10 minutes

Cooking Time: 16 minutes

Servings: 6

Ingredients:

- 1 lb. chicken breast, skinless, boneless, and cut into chunks

- 14.5 oz canned cannellini beans

- 4 cups chicken broth

- 2 cups wild rice

- 1 tbsp Italian seasoning

- 1 small onion, chopped

- 1 tbsp garlic, chopped

- 1 tbsp olive oil

- Pepper

- Salt

Directions:

1. Warm oil into the pot, then put garlic and onion and sauté for 2 minutes.

2. Add chicken and cook for 2 minutes. Add the remaining ingredients and stir well.

3. Cook on high for 12 minutes. Stir well and serve.

Nutrition:

- Calories: 399

- Fat: 6.4 g

- Carbohydrates: 53.4 g

- Sugar: 3 g

- Protein: 31.6 g

- Cholesterol: 50 mg

18. Tasty Greek Rice

Preparation Time: 10 minutes

Cooking Time: 10 minutes

Servings: 6

Ingredients:

- 1 3/4 cup brown rice, rinsed and drained

- 3/4 cup roasted red peppers, chopped

- 1 cup olives, chopped

- 1 tsp dried oregano

- 1 tsp Greek seasoning

- 1 3/4 cup vegetable broth

- 2 tbsp olive oil

- Salt

Directions:

1. Put rice in a pot with olive oil and cook for 5 minutes.

2. Add the remaining ingredients except for red peppers and olives and stir well—cook on high for 5 minutes.

3. Add red peppers and olives and stir well. Serve and enjoy.

Nutrition:

- Calories: 285

- Fat: 9.1 g

- Carbohydrates: 45.7 g

- Sugar: 1.2 g

- Protein: 6 g

- Cholesterol: 0 mg

19.   Bulgur Salad

Preparation Time: 10 minutes

Cooking Time: 1 minute

Servings: 2

Ingredients:

- ½ cup bulgur wheat

- 1/4 cup fresh parsley, chopped

- 1 tbsp fresh mint, chopped

- 1/3 cup feta cheese, crumbled

- 2 tbsp fresh lemon juice

- 2 tbsp olives, chopped

- 1/4 cup olive oil

- ½ cup tomatoes, chopped

- 1/3 cup cucumber, chopped

- ½ cup water

- Salt

Directions:

1. Add the bulgur wheat, water, and salt into the instant pot. Cook on high for 1 minute.

2. Transfer bulgur wheat to the mixing bowl. Put the rest of the ingredients in the bowl and mix well. Serve and enjoy.

Nutrition:

- Calories: 430

- Fat: 32.2 g

- Carbohydrates: 31.5 g

- Sugar: 3 g

- Protein: 8.9 g

- Cholesterol: 22 mg

20.   Perfect Herb Rice

Preparation Time: 10 minutes

Cooking Time: 4 minutes

Servings: 4

Ingredients:

- 1 cup brown rice, rinsed

- 1 tbsp olive oil 1 ½ cups water

- ½ cup fresh mix herbs, chopped

- 1 tsp salt

Directions:

1. Put all the ingredients into the pot and stir well. Cook on high for 4 minutes. Stir well and serve.

Nutrition:

- Calories: 264 Fat: 9.9 g Carbohydrates: 36.7 g

- Sugar: 0.4 g Protein: 7.3 g Cholesterol: 0 mg

21. Cherry, Apricot, and Pecan Brown Rice Bowl

Preparation Time: 15 minutes

Cooking Time: 61 minutes

Servings: 2

Ingredients:

- 2 tablespoons olive oil

- 2 green onions, sliced

- ½ cup of brown rice

- 1 cup low -sodium chicken stock

- 2 tablespoons dried cherries

- 4 dried apricots, chopped

- 2 tablespoons pecans, toasted and chopped

- Sea salt

- Ground pepper

Directions:

1. Warm-up the olive oil in a medium saucepan over medium-high heat until shimmering.

2. Add the green onions and sauté for 1 minute or until fragrant. Add the rice. Stir to mix well, then pour in the chicken stock.

3. Bring to a boil. Reduce the heat to low. Cover and simmer for 50 minutes or until the brown rice is soft.

4. Add the cherries, apricots, and pecans, and simmer for 10 more minutes or until the fruits are tender.

5. Pour them in a large serving bowl—fluff with a fork. Put sea salt plus ground pepper. Serve immediately.

Nutrition:

- Calories: 451 Fat: 25.9g

- Protein: 8.2g Carbs: 50.4g Fiber: 4.6g Sodium: 122mg

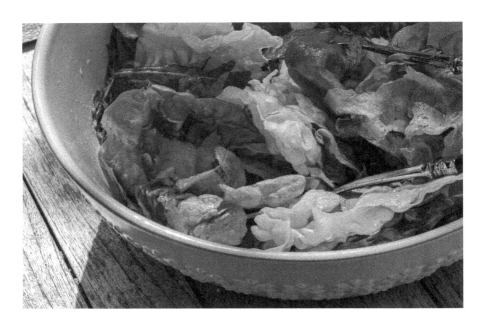

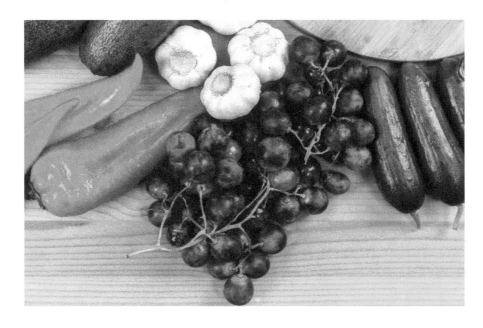

CHAPTER 6:

Here Are the Main Courses of Meat That Will Make You the Master Chef of Your Circle of Friends

22. Italian Pork Loin

Preparation Time: 15 minutes

Cooking Time: 2 hours & 20 minutes

Servings: 2

Ingredients:

- 1-40 ounces trimmed pork loin

- 1 teaspoon of kosher salt

- 3 cloves crushed and peeled garlic

- 2 tablespoons of extra-virgin olive oil

- 2 tablespoons fresh rosemary, chopped

- 1 tablespoon lemon zest, freshly grated

- 3/4 cup of dry vermouth (or substitute with white wine)

- 2 tablespoons of white wine vinegar

Directions:

1. Tie the loin with a kitchen string on two sides and the middle so it will not flatten.

2. Mash the salt and garlic to make a paste. Stir in the other ingredients except for the vermouth and the vinegar. Rub the mixture all over the loin and refrigerate without cover for an hour.

3. Roast loin at a preheated temperature of 375 F, turning it over once or twice for 40 to 50 minutes. Move it into a cutting board and let it cool for 10 minutes.

4. While cooling, pour the vermouth and vinegar into your roasting pan over medium-high temperature. Simmer for 2 to 4 minutes, scraping off the brown bits and reducing the liquid to half.

5. Remove string and slice the roast. Add excess juice to the sauce and serve.

Nutrition:

- Calories: 182

- Carbohydrates: 0.6 g

- Fiber: 0.1 g

- Fats: 8.3 g

- Sodium: 149 mg

- Protein: 20.6 g

23. Mediterranean Chili Beef

Preparation Time: 15 minutes

Cooking Time: 25 minutes

Servings: 4

Ingredients:

- 8 ounces lean ground beef

- 4 minced garlic cloves

- 3/4 teaspoon of salt, divided

- 1/4 teaspoon pepper

- 3 teaspoons of olive oil, divided

- 1 medium sliced red onion

- 2 medium zucchinis, sliced

- 1 medium-size green pepper

- 1-28 ounces can dice tomatoes, undrained

- 1 teaspoon of red wine vinegar

- 1 teaspoon of dried basil

- 1 teaspoon of dried thyme

Directions:

1. Sauté beef in ¼-teaspoon salt, garlic, pepper, and a teaspoon of oil over medium heat until the beef turns brown. Drain and remove. Keep warm.

2. Using the same skillet, pour the remaining oil and sauté onion. Add zucchini and green pepper and stir-cook for 4 to 6 minutes until crisp-tender.

3. Stir in the remaining ingredients. Add beef and cook until heated through—suggested serving over pasta or brown rice.

Nutrition:

- Calories: 204 Carbohydrates: 18 g

- Fiber: 6 g Fats: 9 g

- Sodium: 739 mg rotein: 15 g

24. Cherry Sauce Meatballs

Preparation Time: 30 minutes

Cooking Time: 15 minutes

Servings: 42

Ingredients:

- 1 cup bread crumbs, seasoned

- 1 small chopped onion

- 1 large lightly beaten egg

- 3 minced garlic cloves

- 1 teaspoon salt

- ½ teaspoon pepper

- 16-ounce 90% lean ground beef

- 16-ounce ground pork

Sauce:

- 1-21 ounce can cherry pie filling

- 1/3 cup sherry (or substitute chicken broth)

- 1/3 cup of cider vinegar

- 1/4 cup of steak sauce

- 2 tablespoons of brown sugar

- 2 tablespoons soy sauce, reduced-sodium

- 1 teaspoon honey

Directions:

1. Preheat your oven to 400 F.

2. Mix the first six ingredients and mix well. Add the ground meat and mix thoroughly. Shape the mixture into 1-inch balls. Arrange in a shallow baking pan over a greased rack.

3. Bake for 11 to 13 minutes or until cooked through. Drain juice on a paper towel.

4. In a large-size saucepan, combine all sauce ingredients. Boil the sauce over medium heat. Simmer uncovered within 2 to 3 minutes or until it thickens.

5. Add the meatballs stir gently until heated through.

Nutrition:

- Calories: 76

- Carbohydrates: 7 g

- Fiber: 0 g

- Fats: 3 g Sodium: 169 mg

- Protein: 5 g

25. Pork in Blue Cheese Sauce

Preparation Time: 15 minutes **Cooking Time:** 30 minutes

Servings: 6

Ingredients:

- 2 pounds pork center-cut loin roast, boneless and cut into 6 pieces 1 tablespoon coconut amino

- 6 ounces blue cheese 1/3 cup heavy cream

- 1/3 cup port wine

- 1/3 cup roasted vegetable broth, preferably homemade

- 1 teaspoon dried hot Chile flake

- 1 teaspoon dried rosemary

- 1 tablespoon lard

- 1 shallot, chopped

- 2 garlic cloves, chopped

- Salt

- cracked black peppercorns

Directions:

1. Rub each piece of the pork with salt, black peppercorns, and rosemary.

2. Melt the lard in a saucepan over a moderately high flame. Sear the pork on all sides for about 15 minutes; set aside.

3. Cook the shallot and garlic until they've softened. Add in port wine to scrape up any brown bits from the bottom.

4. Adjust to medium-low, add in the remaining ingredients; continue to simmer until the sauce has thickened and reduced.

Nutrition:

- Calories: 34 Fat: 18.9g Carbs: 1.9g

- Protein: 40.3g Fiber: 0.3g

26.   Mississippi Pulled Pork

Preparation Time: 15 minutes

Cooking Time: 6 hours

Servings: 4

Ingredients:

- 1 ½ pound pork shoulder

- 1 tablespoon liquid smoke sauce

- 1 teaspoon chipotle powder

- Au Jus gravy seasoning packet

- 2 onions, cut into wedges

- Kosher salt

- ground black pepper

Directions:

1. Mix the liquid smoke sauce, chipotle powder, Au Jus gravy seasoning packet, salt, and pepper. Massage the spice mixture into the pork on all sides.

2. Wrap in plastic wrap and let it marinate in your refrigerator for 3 hours.

3. Prepare your grill for indirect heat. Place the pork butt roast on the grate over a drip pan and top with onions; cover the grill and cook for about 6 hours.

4. Transfer the pork to a cutting board. Now, shred the meat into bite-sized pieces using two forks.

Nutrition:

- Calories: 350

- Fat: 11g

- Carbs: 5g

- Protein: 53.6g

- Fiber: 2.2g

27. Spicy and Cheesy Turkey Dip

Preparation Time: 15 minutes

Cooking Time: 25 minutes

Servings: 4

Ingredients:

- 1 Fresno chili pepper, deveined and minced

- 1 ½ cups Ricotta cheese, creamed, 4% fat, softened

- 1/4 cup sour cream

- 1 tablespoon butter, room temperature

- 1 shallot, chopped

- 1 teaspoon garlic, pressed

- 1-pound ground turkey

- ½ cup goat cheese, shredded

- Salt and black pepper, to taste

- 1 ½ cups Gruyere, shredded

Directions:

1. Dissolve the butter in a frying pan over a moderately high flame. Now, sauté the onion and garlic until they have softened.

2. Stir in the ground turkey and continue to cook until it is no longer pink.

3. Transfer the sautéed mixture to a lightly greased baking dish. Add in Ricotta, sour cream, goat cheese, salt, pepper, and chili pepper.

4. Top with the shredded Gruyere cheese. Bake at 350 degrees F within 20 minutes in the preheated oven or until hot and bubbly on top.

Nutrition:

- Calories: 284 Fat: 19g

- Carbs: 3.2g Protein: 26g

- Fiber: 1.6g

28.   Turkey Chorizo with Bok Choy

Preparation Time: 15 minutes **Cooking Time:** 50 minutes

Servings: 4

Ingredients:

- 4 mild turkey Chorizo, sliced

- ½ cup full-fat milk

- 6 ounces Gruyere cheese, preferably freshly grated

- 1 yellow onion, chopped

- Coarse salt ground black pepper

- 1-pound Bok choy, tough stem ends trimmed

- 1 cup cream of mushroom soup

- 1 tablespoon lard, room temperature

Directions:

1. Melt the lard in a non-stick skillet over a moderate flame; cook the Chorizo sausage for about 5 minutes,

occasionally stirring to ensure even cooking; reserve.

2. Add in the onion, salt, pepper, Bok choy, and cream of mushroom soup. Continue to cook for 4 minutes longer or until the vegetables have softened.

3. Put the batter into a lightly oiled casserole dish. Top with the reserved Chorizo.

4. In a mixing bowl, thoroughly combine the milk and cheese. Pour the cheese mixture over the sausage.

5. Cover with foil and bake at 36degrees F for about 35 minutes.

Nutrition:

- Calories: 18
- Fat: 12g
- Carbs: 2.6g
- Protein: 9.4g
- Fiber: 1g

29.   Za'atar Chicken Tenders

Preparation Time: 5 minutes

Cooking Time: 15 minutes

Servings: 4

Ingredients:

- Olive oil cooking spray

- 1-pound chicken tenders

- 1½ tablespoons za'atar

- ½ teaspoon kosher salt

- ¼ teaspoon freshly ground black pepper

Directions:

1. Preheat the oven to 450°F. Lightly spray with olive oil cooking spray.

2. In a large bowl, combine the chicken, za'atar, salt, and black pepper. Mix well, covering the chicken tenders fully. Arrange in a single sheet on the baking sheet and

bake for 15 minutes, turning the chicken over once midway through cooking.

Nutrition:

- Calories: 145

- Total Fat: 4g

- Cholesterol: 83mg

- Total Carbohydrates: 0g

- Fiber: 0g

CHAPTER 7:

Bring the Blue Sea of the Mediterranean to Your Table with Fantastic Fish and Seafood Dishes

30. Grilled Salmon with Lemon and Wine

Preparation Time: 10 minutes

Cooking Time: 10 minutes

Servings: 4

Ingredients:

- 1 big lemon

- 1 ½ cup of olive oil

- ½ tsp. pepper

- 3 tsp of vegetable oil

- 4 of 6 oz of salmon fillets

- 1 tsp. lime zest

- 1 ½ tbsp. salt

Directions:

1. Prepare the grill and rub the fillets with oil.

2. Put lime zest, lemon zest, salt, and pepper on both sides of the fillets.

3. Brush oil on the grill, put the salmon and the fillets on the grill, and allow it to grill for about 7 minutes. Turn it to the other side and grill for about 3 minutes.

4. The salmon can now be served with lemon wedges.

Nutrition:

- Calories: 270 Carbs: 11.5g

- Fat: 14.2g

- Protein: 28.1g

31.   Olive Oil Poached Cod

Preparation Time: 5 minutes

Cooking Time: 10 minutes

Servings: 4

Ingredients:

- 2 tsp of lemon juice

- 4 of 6 oz of cod fillets

- 3 cups of olive oil

- 1 tsp of lemon zest

- 1 tbsp of salt

Directions:

1. Wash the fillets and put them on a paper towel.

2. Put oil inside a big pot, add the fish's fillets to poach for about 6 minutes, or the fish color changes opaque.

3. Take the fish out of the oil and add salt to it. Put some of the left-over warm oil on the fish, add lemon juice with it. Add zest by sprinkling. It is ready to be served.

Nutrition:

- Calories: 305
- Carbs: 10g
- Fat: 15g
- Protein: 31g

32.   Pistachio-Crusted Halibut

Preparation Time: 15 minutes

Cooking Time: 20 minutes

Servings: 4

Ingredients:

- 4 (6-oz) halibut fillet with skin removed

- ½ cup shelled unsalted pistachios (chopped)

- 4 tsp fresh parsley (chopped)

- 1 cup bread crumbs

- ¼ cup extra-virgin olive oil

- 2 tsp grated orange zest

- 1 tsp. grated lime zest

- ½ tsp. pepper

- 4 tsp of Dijon mustard

- 1½ of salt

Directions:

1. Preheat the oven to 4000F.

2. In the food processor, add pistachio, zest, bread crumbs, parsley, and oil. Pulse until the ingredients are well combined.

3. Rinse the fish and pat dry with a paper towel. Season the fillet with salt and pepper.

4. Brush the fish with mustard and divide the pistachio mix evenly with some on top of the fish. Press down the mixture to allow the crust to adhere.

5. Lining the baking sheet with crusted paper, arrange the crusted fish, and bake for 20minutes or until the fillet is golden brown. Leave for 5 minutes to cool, then

Nutrition:

- Calories: 231 Carbs: 31.5g

- Protein: 5.8g Fat: g

33. Red Mullet Savaro Style

Preparation Time: 20 minutes

Cooking Time: 15 minutes

Servings: 4

Ingredients:

- 4(½-pound) red mullet (cleaned, scaled, and gutted)

- 2 tee-spoon of salt

- 2/3 cup of olive oil

- 2 tbsps. of rosemary

- 8 cloves of finely diced garlic

- 2/3 cup of red wine vinegar

Directions:

1. Massage the fish with salt and leave for 20 minutes.

2. Mix with flour and set aside. Add 1/3 cup of oil to the frying pan and heat over medium-high heat until it is hot; fry each fish 4-5 minutes per side. Set aside

3. Pour the rest of the oil into another frying pan and add rosemary; fry until it turns an olive color, then remove from the oil.

4. Add garlic to the oil and stir until it turns golden. Add the vinegar and stir until the sauce thickens and is bittersweet. Pour the source over the fish and serve.

Nutrition:

- Calories: 150

- Carbs: 2.1g

- Fat: 8g

- Protein: 25g

34. Spinach-Stuffed Sole

Preparation Time: 5 minutes

Cooking Time: 20 minutes

Servings: 4

Ingredients:

- 4 (6-oz) of sole fillets

- 4 scallions with ends trimmed and sliced

- A 1-pound package of frozen spinach (thawed)

- 1 tsp of salt 3tsps. of chopped fennel

- ½ tsp pepper 1tsp sweet paprika

- 2 tbsps. of lemon

Directions:

1. Preheat the oven to 4000F

2. Put a small pan on medium heat, then add 2 tbsp of oil and heat for 3osonds.

3. Add the scallion and cook for 3-4 minutes; allow it to cool.

4. In a bowl, add scallion, spinach, pepper, ½ tsp of salt, and ¼ tsp of pepper. Mix the ingredients

5. Rinse and dry the fillet with a paper towel. Massage the fish with oil and sprinkle with pepper, paprika, and 2 tbsp of lemon.

6. Spread the spinach fillings on the fillets, roll up each fillet starting from the wide-angle and secure each fillet with toothpicks.

7. Bake for 15-20 minutes. Remove the toothpick and sprinkle with lemon zest. Serve immediately

Nutrition:

- Calories: 174 Carb: 1g

- Fat: 6g

- Protein: 39g

35.   Grilled Sardines

Preparation Time: 5 minutes

Cooking Time: 15 minutes

Servings: 4

Ingredients:

- 2 pounds of fresh sardine (clean gutted and scaled with the head removed)

- 2 tsp. of salt

- 3 tbsps. of vegetable oil

- ¾ tsp. of pepper

- 1½ tsp. of dried oregano

- 3 tbsps. of lemon juice

- ½ cup of extra-virgin olive oil (divided)

Directions:

1. Preheat your grill to a medium-high temperature.

2. Rinse the sardine and pat dry with a towel paper, then rub on both sides with olive oil. Sprinkle both sides with pepper and salt.

3. Wipe the grill surface with oil. Place each sardine on the grill and grill for 2-3 minutes; while grilling, drizzle the sardine with olive oil and lemon juice.

4. Sprinkle with oregano and serve.

Nutrition:

- Calories: 231

- Carb: 0.6g

- Protein: 26g

- Fats: 13.6g

36.   Pickled & Preserved Octopus in Olive Oil

Preparation Time: 20 minutes

Cooking Time: 5 hours

Servings: 6

Ingredients:

- 2-lbs large octopus tentacles

- 10-cloves garlic, peeled (divided)

- 3-cups olive oil

- 1-tsp white peppercorns

- 3-pcs fresh bay leaves

- ½-cup lemon juice

- 1-cup verjuice or crabapple juice

- 1-tsp dried Greek oregano (rigatoni)

- ¾-cup water

- Flat-leaf parsley leaves, torn black olives, and thinly sliced cucumber for garnish

Directions:

1. Preheat your oven to 375 °F. To pickle or make a confit octopus, put the octopus, half of the garlic cloves, olive oil, peppercorns, and a piece of bay leaf in a baking dish. Cover the dish tightly with aluminum foil. Put the dish in the preheated oven. Bake for 5 hours until tender.

2. Take away the dish from the oven, and let it cool completely in the oil. Reserve 1-cup of the confit oil and set aside.

3. Place the confit octopus after that is the reserved confit. Use oil in an 8-quart sterilized jar.

4. Then pour in the lemon juice and verjuice.

5. Next, add the oregano and the remaining garlic cloves and bay leaves. Pour in the water, and seal the jar with its lid. Set the sealed jar aside in a cool and dark place,

turning the jar every couple of hours for 6 hours to pickle.

6. Remove the pickled octopus from the jar. Slice the octopus into large pieces, and then serve with the parsley, olives, and cucumber garnish.

Nutrition:

- Calories: 454

- Total Fats: 35.6g

- Dietary Fiber: 0.4g

- Carbohydrates: 6.1g

- Protein: 28.9g

37. Chunky Crabmeat in Tortilla Tostadas

Preparation Time: 15 minutes

Cooking Time: 15 minutes

Servings: 6

Ingredients:

- 6-pcs whole corn tortilla tostadas

- 2-tbsp olive oil 4-tbsp red onion, minced

- 2-tsp garlic, minced 2-tsp cilantro, minced

- 1¼-cup tomatoes, diced and drained of liquid

- 2-cups crab meat, cooked

- 1/3-cup lettuce, shredded

- 3½-tbsp red bell pepper, chopped

- 1-oz. lemon juice ¼-cup olives 2-oz. salsa

Directions:

1. Preheat your oven to 350 °F. Bake the tortillas for 10 minutes until crisp.

2. Meanwhile, heat the olive oil in a pan placed over medium-high heat and sauté the onion for 3 minutes until tender. Add the garlic, cilantro, tomatoes, and crab meat, Cook for 5 minutes. Set aside.

3. Combine the lettuce, bell pepper, lemon juice, and olives in a mixing bowl. Mix well until thoroughly combined.

4. Divide the vegetable mixture evenly between the tortillas. Then top each tortilla with the crab mixture.

5. Serve with salsa.

Nutrition:

- Calories: 90

- Total Fats: 2g

- Dietary Fiber: 1g

- Carbohydrates: 4g

- Protein: 14g

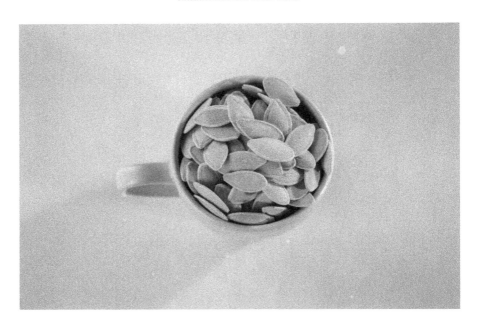

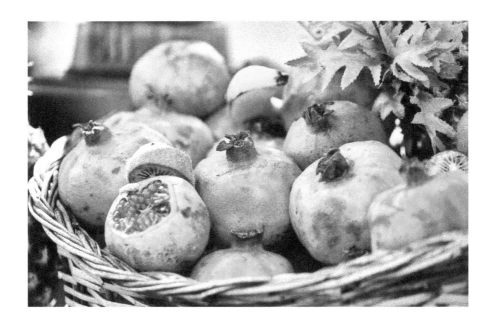

CHAPTER 8:

Prepare Delicious Salads in Minutes

38.   Herbed Chicken Salad Greek Style

Preparation Time: 5 minutes

Cooking Time: 0 minutes

Servings: 6

Ingredients:

- ¼ cup or 1 oz crumbled feta cheese

- ½ tsp garlic powder

- ½ tsp salt

- ¾ tsp black pepper, divided

- 1 cup grape tomatoes, halved

- 1 cup peeled and chopped English cucumbers

- 1 cup plain fat-free yogurt

- 1-pound boneless chicken breast, slice into 1-inch cubes

- 1 tsp bottled minced garlic

- 1 tsp ground oregano

- 2 tsp sesame seed paste or tahini

- 5 tsp fresh lemon juice, divided

- Six pitted kalamata olives, halved

- 8 cups chopped romaine lettuce

- Cooking spray

Directions:

1. In a bowl, mix ¼ tsp salt, ½ tsp pepper, garlic powder, and oregano. Then on medium-high heat, place a skillet and coat with cooking spray and sauté together with

the spice mixture and chicken until chicken is cooked. Before transferring to bowl, drizzle with juice.

2. In a small bowl, mix the following: garlic, tahini, yogurt, ¼ tsp pepper, ¼ tsp salt, and tsp juice thoroughly.

3. In another bowl, mix olives, tomatoes, cucumber, and lettuce.

4. To serve the salad, place 2 ½ cups of lettuce mixture on a plate, topped with ½ cup chicken mixture, 3 tbsp yogurt mixture, and 1 tbsp of cheese.

Nutrition:

- Calories per serving: 170.1

- Fat: 3.7g

- Protein: 20.7g

- Carbs: 13.5g

39. Roasted Bell Pepper Salad with Anchovy Dressing

Preparation Time: 5 minutes

Cooking Time: 20 minutes

Servings: 4

Ingredients:

- Eight roasted red bell peppers, sliced

- Two tablespoons pine nuts

- 1 cup cherry tomatoes, halved

- Two tablespoons chopped parsley

- Four anchovy fillets

- One lemon, juiced

- One garlic clove

- One tablespoon extra-virgin olive oil

- Salt and pepper to taste

Directions:

1. Combine the anchovy fillets, lemon juice, garlic, and olive oil in a mortar and mix them well.

2. Mix the rest of the ingredients in a salad bowl, then drizzle in the dressing.

3. Serve the salad as fresh as possible.

Nutrition:

- Calories: 81

- Fat: 7.0g

- Protein: 2.4g

- Carbohydrates: 4.0g

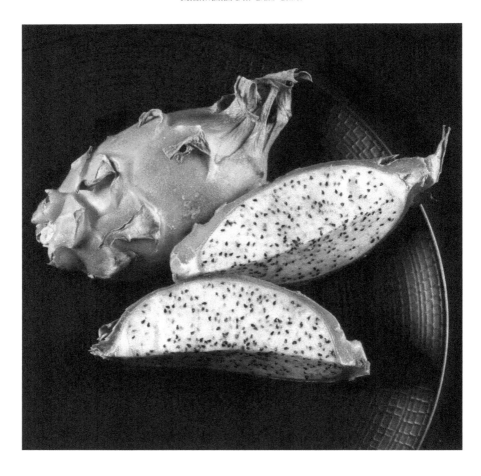

CHAPTER 9:

Preparation of Desserts That Will Make

Your Guests' Mouth Water

40.   Strawberries Cream

Preparation Time: 10 minutes

Cooking Time: 20 minutes

Servings: 4

Ingredients:

- ½ cup stevia

- 2 pounds strawberries, chopped

- 1 cup almond milk

- Zest of 1 lemon, grated

- ½ cup heavy cream

- Three egg yolks whisked

Directions:

1. Heat a pan with the milk over medium-high heat, add the stevia and the rest of the ingredients. Whisk well, simmer for 20 minutes, divide into cups and serve cold.

Nutrition:

- Calories: 152

- Fat: 4.4 g

- Fiber: 5.5 g

- Carbs: 5.1 g

- Protein: 0.8 g

Conclusion

Thank you for making it through to the end of the Mediterranean diet. This diet is so beautiful in nature that it is hard not to fall in love with it. Learning about this diet is an absolute requirement of life.

If I have managed to spark your interest, then the Mediterranean diet is waiting for you. The Mediterranean diet is waiting for you to call its own. It is hard to resist the enticement of exploring the Mediterranean diet and having a wonderful Mediterranean life. The happiest times in my life I have spent away from the Mediterranean diet, and it is about time I get back there. The Mediterranean diet is truly magical, and the way of life we should all follow as it is most satisfying and fulfilling.

If you have or have not been following the Mediterranean diet, then you should do yourself a favor and start. Start eating right and enjoying life. Do so, and you shall only be happy. Stop avoiding the Mediterranean diet and jump in.

The Mediterranean diet is a diet that allows you to spend every single day eating wonderful food. The amazing fact about it is that it has ruined your taste for any other food available. You simply can't be happy until you have a good meal that includes the Mediterranean diet.

If you have already adopted the Mediterranean diet, then take time to take a step back and look around you. You should see people of all shapes and sizes having a wonderful life. They must be following the Mediterranean diet. There is no other possible conclusion.

The Mediterranean diet isn't only an approach to shied weight; however, it is an approach to transform you completely, and in doing as such, dragging out it. The medical advantages are perpetual, particularly when they are joined with work out, making this nourishment experience something unquestionably worth investigating. The primary concern is — the individuals who are on this eating regimen have lower death rates than the individuals who are not, which is reason enough to try it out. In the event that you have a past filled with coronary illness in your family, you truly can't stand to proceed in a similar way, and now you have another option.

If you have tried the Mediterranean diet, you may be thinking about going back to old habits. Don't do it. It may make sense at that moment, but you will regret it later as it never does any good. Continue down the path of the Mediterranean diet. It is a path that winds endlessly in circles. You will never regret following the Mediterranean diet and enjoying wonderful meals while you think about your meals. The memories of them will never go away. If you have adopted the Mediterranean diet, you should know that there is a whole world out there with far more to offer than what you are currently savoring. The world of taste is so big that you will always be hungry for more. So, when a thought comes into your head, you should make a note to try the Mediterranean diet in more than just your head. Follow it through.

CPSIA information can be obtained
at www.ICGtesting.com
Printed in the USA
BVHW062320250321
603415BV00005B/576

9 781802 233520